Prebiotics
And
Probiotics

J. Anthony von Fraunhofer
MSc, PhD, FRSC
Professor Emeritus
University of Maryland, Baltimore

DEDICATION

Susan, the light of my life

CONTENTS

1 INTRODUCTION

Prebiotics, probiotics and antibiotics are all compounds that are ingested to achieve certain effects within the body. Prebiotics are food ingredients that are not digested by intestinal enzymes and so reach the colon mostly intact where they are digested by the colonic microflora. Probiotics are beneficial or "friendly" bacteria normally present in the mouth and the intestines, and they help maintain a healthy internal environment. Antibiotics are natural or synthetic agents that control pathogens within the body but, along with many other therapeutic agents, they also may affect the bacteria within the digestive tract. Such effects may be beneficial or adverse, depending upon the mode of action of the antimicrobial agent. Antibiotics, however, will not be discussed here because they are a prescription medication and, as such, are beyond the scope of this book.

The digestive tract is discussed in Chapter 1 but a few words by way of introduction might be useful here. The digestive tract traverses the entire body, starting at the mouth and ending at the anus. The stomach is the reservoir that collects ingested food and liquids and, after digestion with stomach acids and some enzymes, the residue is ejected in small amounts into the small bowel, a structure that is over 20 feet (6 meters) in length. The small bowel is supplied with digestive juices and enzymes from the liver and pancreas and these act together to digest food. After digestion, the food constituents, i.e., the carbohydrates, minerals, vitamins, amino acids, fats and calories, are absorbed into the blood stream and carried throughout the body.

The residue from the small bowel flows into the colon, a structure approximately 5 feet (1.5 meter) in length, after which it is moved to the rectum and evacuated. The colon resorbs fluid as well as other components and compacts feces so that until comparatively recently, it was regarded as a waste depot for food residues despite the fact that it is extensively colonized by bacteria. Now it is recognized that some of the bacteria in the gut have a variety of health benefits, including assisting in absorption of nutrients, emitting short-chain fatty acids that help build the colon wall and drive out bad bacteria. Beneficial bacteria also appear to prevent hypersensitivity reactions such as allergies and asthma as well as reduce triglycerides within the blood. The colon also is populated by numerous species of bacteria that have less desirable effects and may be pathogenic; these bacterial species include *Escherichia coli (E. coli)*, *Salmonella* and *Clostridium difficile (C. diff)* and they actively compete with beneficial bacteria in the colonization of the colon. If the bad bacteria

11

predominate, they will cause a variety of adverse effects.

High concentrations of "bad" bacteria can cause severe diarrhea, as is the case with *C. diff,* while the toxic and sometimes fatal effects caused by food contamination by *Salmonella* and *E. coli* are well known. Other less desirable but less toxic bacteria in the gut will digest any sulfur present in foodstuffs to emit hydrogen sulfide (H_2S) which not only appears to be related to the prevalence of ulcerative colitis but also confers the rotten egg smell on flatus.

This book discusses the role of prebiotics and probiotics in maintaining systemic health (i.e. affecting the entire body) as well as addressing the multiplicity of microbial species that exist within the body. Although prebiotics and probiotics are discussed in separate chapters, these divisions are somewhat artificial because these agents are interrelated. The objective of this book is to show the interrelationship between these active agents within the biosystem and to indicate how health is determined and controlled by these interactions.

Finally, a glossary of terms is provided at the back of the book for easy reference to the many technical terms that inevitably crop up in any discussion of health-related subjects.

J. A. von Fraunhofer
Ocala, FL
September, 2012

J. A. von FRAUNHOFER

1. THE DIGESTIVE TRACT

In order to appreciate the role of prebiotics and probiotics in human health, it is important to have some understanding of the anatomy and physiology of the gastrointestinal (GI) system. This chapter provides a basic guide to the GI system and its various components; however, the interested reader is advised to consult specialized works on anatomy and physiology for more detailed information.

Anatomy

The alimentary or digestive tract traverses the entire body, starting at the mouth and ending at the anus. The alimentary tract, shown schematically in Figure 1.1, includes the mouth, pharynx, esophagus, stomach, ileum (small intestine), colon (large intestine), the rectum and the anus.

Figure 1.1 *The human digestive system*

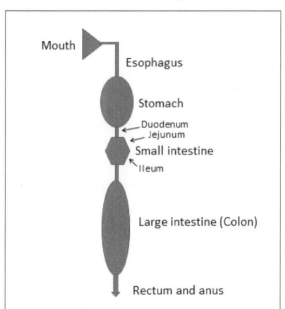

The diagram shows the alimentary system as a straight connection between mouth and anus but within the body, the large intestine follows a quasi-rectangular path that surrounds the small intestine.

Food intake and digestion

The entry portal to the digestive system is the oral cavity or mouth. Ideally the mouth has 32 teeth although the actual number present is often less than that. Teeth may be missing for numerous reasons, including decay (dental caries), periodontitis (gum disease), extractions to ease crowding, or simply because some teeth are congenitally missing. Regardless of the reason, missing teeth is not necessarily a health problem. The World Health Organization has indicated that a functional, esthetic natural dentition only requires a minimum of 20 teeth. Likewise, the dental literature indicates that dental arches comprising only the anterior and premolar regions (i.e. few or no molar teeth) meet the requirements of a functional dentition.

The human dentition comprises different types of teeth, all of which have a specific role with regard to the intake of food. The anterior (front) teeth are used for incising or cutting into foodstuffs whereas the posterior (back) teeth chew (masticate) food. The oral cavity also contains various glands that supply the mouth with saliva, the latter containing certain proteins and enzymes that initiate the digestive processes during mastication. Saliva also performs other essential functions, notably helping rinse foodstuffs from the teeth, maintaining the pH or acidity in the mouth close to neutrality to reduce acid attack on the teeth, and helping to remineralize the teeth to offset damage caused by acidic attack.

The oral cavity contains high concentrations of multiple species of micro-organisms, many of which are beneficial whereas others are potentially harmful. The concentration and variety of bacterial species will vary depending upon diet, oral hygiene and the presence of prostheses (e.g. dentures).

After mastication, food and liquids are passed through the esophagus into the stomach where ingested food and liquids are collected. After interacting with stomach acids and selective enzymes, the partially digested material, a thick, semifluid mass known as chyme, is passed in small amounts into the small intestine, a structure that is over 20 feet (6 meters) in length. The small intestine is supplied with digestive juices and enzymes from its intrinsic glands as well as from the two major extrinsic glands of the digestive system, the liver and pancreas, and these juices and enzymes all act together to digest food.

The small intestine

The small intestine (small bowel) is comprised of the duodenum at the upper end, a middle section or jejunum and the ileum at the lower end. Although there is no sharp demarcation between the jejunum and the ileum, there are some differences between the two in that the ileum is paler in color and has a lesser diameter. The jejunum and the ileum are suspended by mesentery which gives the small bowel great mobility within the abdomen. The entire length of the small intestine is wrapped by smooth muscle which helps transport food through the bowel by a pulsing process known as peristalsis. In contrast to the acidic (low pH) conditions of the stomach, the pH in the small intestine is usually between 7 and 8, that is, neutral to weakly alkaline. The mucous membrane inner surfaces of the jejunum and ileum have a number of folds and these are covered in projecting filaments (villi) which greatly increase the surface area and facilitate absorption of nutrients from the gut. These nutrients include fructose, amino acids, small peptides, vitamins and most glucose molecules. Small lymph vessels also are present within the villi and these help absorption of fatty acids and glycerol, the digestion products of fat. The villi in the jejunum are much longer than those in the duodenum or ileum.

The primary function of the ileum, the final section of the small intestine, is to absorb vitamin B12, bile salts and residual digestion products not absorbed by the jejunum. The very large surface area of the ileum facilitates the adsorption of enzymes and digestion products. The diffuse neuroendocrine system (DNES) cells lining the ileum contain protease and carbohydrase enzymes, notably gastrin, secretin and cholecystokinin; these enzymes are responsible for the final stages of protein and carbohydrate digestion and are also present in the cytoplasm of the epithelial cells. The villi lining the ileum (and jejunum) contain large numbers of capillaries which transport the amino acids and glucose produced by digestion to the hepatic portal vein and the liver.

Overall, the digestion process results in individual food components, notably carbohydrates, minerals, vitamins, amino acids, and fats, being absorbed into the blood stream and carried throughout the body.

The residues from the small bowel are moved by muscle contraction (peristalsis) into the large bowel (intestine) or colon, a structure approximately 5 feet (1.5 meter) in length. Ultimately, the residue is moved to the rectum and evacuated. Until comparatively recently, the colon commonly was regarded as a waste depository for food residues despite being extensively colonized by bacteria. It is now recognized that the colonic microorganisms (the flora or microorganisms present within the colon) are essential components in the re-absorption of water.

Microflora of the GI tract

Some 80% of the cells of the immune system reside within the small and large intestines. Under normal circumstances, the gastrointestinal tract contains a balanced number of beneficial and potentially harmful bacteria. This collection of micro-organisms is known as the normal (or natural) microflora. It was also noted above that the oral cavity contains high concentrations of multiple species of micro-organisms.

Due to its acidity, the stomach was previously considered to be sterile. It is now recognized that certain bacteria such as *Helicobacter pylori* are found in large numbers in the stomachs of some individuals. The small and large intestines contain multiple species of Gram positive and Gram negative rods and cocci (see Chapter 2). The health benefits of these bacteria include absorption of nutrients, facilitation of calcium and magnesium absorption, and generation of short-chain fatty acids which assist in regenerating the colon wall. Further, bacteria also help make vitamin K and maintain the immune system functioning properly. Beneficial bacteria also appear to prevent hypersensitivity reactions such as allergies and asthma as well as reduce triglyceride levels within the blood.

In general, micro-organisms in the proximal (right) side of the colon, known as the ascending colon, grow at a fast rate because of a good supply of nutrients, and the fermentation products of digested nutrients produced by these bacteria include short chain fatty acids that cause a decrease in the pH, i.e. the acidity is increased. Bacteria in the distal (left) side of the colon, the descending colon, have a more restricted nutrient supply and grow more slowly so that the pH approaches neutrality.

The colon also is populated by numerous species of bacteria, some of which may cause disease under certain circumstances. These potential pathogens may actively compete with beneficial bacteria in colonizing the colon and the relative concentrations of beneficial *vs.* pathogenic bacteria can impact health. An example of this is the toxin-producing microorganism, *Clostridium difficile.* When present at low levels, *C. difficile* causes minimal if any side-effects. However, when present at high concentrations this micro-organism can cause life-threatening disease. Some less desirable bacteria in the gut convert sulfur-containing compounds present in foodstuffs to hydrogen sulfide (H_2S), a poisonous gas with an offensive smell. Hydrogen sulfide confers the rotten egg smell on flatus (the gas we emit some time after eating) and has been related to the prevalence of ulcerative colitis.

Healthy people have a proper balance in the numbers and types of intestinal bacteria. However, several factors, including poor diet, natural aging, stress and antibiotic therapy, can upset this delicate balance and, for example, a preponderance of "bad" bacteria can be caused by elevated intestinal pH. Bacterial imbalance that results in an overgrowth or preponderance of bad bacteria and yeast within the gut is known as intestinal dyspepsia.

Ingestible microorganisms (known as probiotics) and agents that can increase their numbers (known as prebiotics) can have a major and often beneficial impact on the human gut and overall (systemic) health. These subjects are discussed in the following chapters.

J. A. von FRAUNHOFER

2. BACTERIA

Most articles (and advertisements) concerning the health benefits of probiotics (and prebiotics) refer to "good" and "bad" bacteria. Likewise, mention is made of bacteria throughout this book. However, such imprecise nomenclature can cause confusion for readers. Accordingly, some discussion of bacteria is provided here so that there is a frame of reference for subsequent comments. Readers are advised to consult monographs on microbiology for more detailed information on bacteria and bacterial species.

Bacteria within the Biosystem

Vast numbers of bacteria exist within the body and are necessary for the overall health and viability of the human biosystem. There are, in fact, over 400 different species of bacteria have been identified in the GI tract, the skin, the vaginal tract and the oral cavity, totaling over 10^{14} bacterial cells. The human body hosts over 10,000 microbial species and their combined weight exceeds 3.3 lb. (1.5 kg). In fact, there are at least ten times more bacterial cells on or in the body than the total number of cells (approximately 10^{13}) that constitute the human body. The indigenous intestinal bacteria perform a variety of functions throughout the alimentary tract and are commensal, that is, they co-exist in a manner that they are not harmful to each other and actually may be beneficial to individual species.

Bacteria

Commonly, reference is made to rods and cocci when bacteria are discussed. A coccus, the plural being cocci, is a type of bacterium (plural being bacteria) that has a spherical or ovoid shape. A cluster of bacteria that has the appearance of a bunch of grapes is designated "staphylococci" and chains of clustered bacteria are entitled "streptococci". Many cocci but certainly not all are pathogenic, causing a variety of diseases such as "strep. throat", pneumonia, meningitis, gonorrhea and rheumatic fever, to name but a few. Rod bacteria, as the name implies, are those microbial species having the shape of a rod.

In microbiology, the term "colony forming unit" or CFU is often used. This refers to a common laboratory procedure in which a small volume of a dilute microbial mixture containing about 100-200 cells is transferred to the center of a culturing medium such as an agar plate and spread evenly over the surface with a sterile bent-glass rod. The number of colonies (i.e., growing clumps of bacteria) should equal the number of viable organisms in the sample. The appearance of the CFUs and their staining characteristics (see later) are used to identify the species under examination.

Finally, a word about nomenclature: it is customary in microbiology to shorten the name of a particular genus or family of bacteria to a single capital letter, usually italicized, with a second word indicating which species is under discussion, e.g. *Escherichia coli* is commonly referred to as *E. coli*, *Escherichia* being the genus and *coli* the species.

Gram-positive and Gram-negative bacteria

Bacterial species are also classified as being Gram-positive or Gram-negative based on the chemical and physical properties of their cell walls. This classification derives from a method of staining of bacteria used for their identification that was developed by Hans C. J. Gram. Gram's staining method primarily detects peptidoglycan in the cell wall. Peptidoglycan is a polymer of amino acids and sugars that forms a mesh-like layer comprising the cell wall. The peptidoglycan layer is much thicker (20-80 nanometers) in Gram-positive bacteria than it is Gram-negative bacteria (7-8 nm).

Gram's staining method takes advantage of this difference in peptidoglycan cell wall layer thickness. In particular, a Gram-positive bacterium will take on a purple/blue color in Gram's Method whereas a Gram-negative bacterium assumes a pink/red color.

The staining process involves four steps. The first step involves applying a stain (crystal violet or gentian violet) to a smear of dead bacteria on a glass slide for one minute, rinsing off the dye and then immersing the slide in a solution of a trapping agent (Gram's iodine). After rinsing, the dyed bacteria are rapidly decolorized in 95% alcohol or acetone and then counterstained with safranin or carbolfuchsin for 30 seconds. Thereafter, the treated slide is rinsed and blotted dry. Gram-positive bacteria retain the violet dye and develop a purple coloration whereas Gram-negative bacteria appear pink in color, i.e. they take on the color of the counterstain. Interestingly, both Gram-positive and Gram-negative micro-organisms are always present in the mouth and microbiologists often take bacterial samples from between their teeth. These are then are placed on the glass slide in order to check that the staining method has worked properly. Carbolfuchsin sometimes is used as the counterstain because it stains anaerobic bacteria more intensely than safranin (anaerobic and aerobic bacteria are discussed below).

Most bacteria can be characterized as Gram-positive or Gram-negative, certain bacterial species, known as Gram-variable, will yield a mixture of purple and pink cells after staining. In other words, there can be Gram-negative staining of Gram-positive bacteria with the same species. This happens with genera (species) having cell membranes that are sensitive to breakdown during cell division (e.g. *Actinomyces*), because the cell membrane peptidoglycan thickness decreases during growth (e.g. *Clostridium*) or sometimes the staining characteristics are affected by the age of the culture that is being tested.

There are certain bacterial species, known as Gram-indeterminate bacteria, which do not respond to Gram staining. These species together with Gram-variable bacteria cannot be classified as either Gram-positive or Gram-negative.

Gram-negative Bacteria

Gram-negative bacteria are generally considered pathogens, that is, they are judged harmful to the host. This is evident from Table 2.1 which lists in alphabetical order, the principal Gram-negative bacteria and their associated disease(s). Nevertheless, most bacteria in the gut are Gram-negative but are not harmful unless transported to other locations in the body.

Significantly contributing to the pathogenicity of Gram-negative bacteria is the structure of the cell wall membrane, the outer portion of which is a complex lipopolysaccharide. The lipid portion of the membrane can act as a endotoxin, that is, a bacterial toxin within the body of the bacterium, which is only released when the bacterium breaks down. If the endotoxin enters the circulatory system and then can reach any part of the body, it can cause pathological effects such as a toxic reaction. In the latter case, the sufferer developing a high temperature (known as a pyrogenic effect), an accelerated respiration rate and low blood pressure, and this sometimes may lead to fatal endotoxic toxic.

Although millions of Gram-negative bacteria are present in the gut intestine, endotoxin released by these bacteria is detoxified and eliminated by the liver in healthy individuals. However, if the level of endotoxin increases beyond that which can be detoxified by the liver and starts spreading through the body, the immune system releases an inflammatory substance and causes the body temperature to rise and fight the infection. High levels of endotoxin in the blood, greater than that

Table 2.1 *Principal Gram-negative bacteria and associated diseases*

Genus	Species	Associated Disease
Bordetella	B. pertussis	Whooping cough
Brucella	Br. abortus	Undulant fever
Escherichia	E. coli	Cystitis, pyelitis, suppuration*
Hemophilus	H. influenza	Meningitis, conjunctivitis, influenza
Klebsiella	K. pneumonia	Pneumonia*
Neisseria	N. meningitides	Cerebrospinal meningitis
Proteus	P. vulgaris	Suppuration
Pseudomonas	P. mallei	Glanders
	P. aeruginosa	Suppuration
Salmonella	S. typhosa	Typhoid fever
Shigella	S. dysenteriae	Bacillary dysentry
	S. paratyphi	Paratyphoid fever, gastroenteritis
Vibrio	V. comma	Cholera
Yersinia	Y. pestis	Plague

(*: Occasionally associated with these species)

controllable by the immune system, ultimately can lead to endotoxic shock.

Although certain antibiotics counteract and work against Gram-negative bacteria, it is essential that the patient complete the prescribed course of antibiotics in order for the antibiotics to work properly and to stop the Gram-negative bacteria from developing resistance to these antibiotics.

Gram-Positive Bacteria

As indicated above, Gram-positive bacteria cell membranes contain peptidoglycan which acquires a violet color on staining and the most important forms of Gram-positive bacteria are bacilli (rod-shaped microorganisms) and cocci (spherical or ovoid in shape). Certain Gram-positive bacteria are pathogenic but many are beneficial to the human body, i.e. they are the "good" bacteria. Most, but not all, Gram-positive bacteria are considered non-pathogenic.

Beneficial Gram-positive bacteria

Lactobacilli are Gram-positive, rod-shaped bacteria that are found as single cells or chains and are present in the flora (i.e. collections of bacterial species occurring or adapted to living in a specific environment) of the mouth and the vagina These bacteria produce lactic acid as part of their metabolic activity. Certain species are involved in the production of yogurt, sour cream and buttermilk. A number of *Lactobacillus* species are the principal components of probiotics formulations.

Bifidobacteria are Gram-positive anaerobic bacteria that are one of the major genera of bacteria making up the colon flora in mammals. They are ubiquitous in the gastrointestinal tract, vagina and mouth. Before the 1960s, *Bifidobacterium* species were collectively referred to as "*Lactobacillus bifidus*" but this terminology has now been abandoned. Some *Bifidobacterium* species and/or strains are considered important probiotics and are used in

37

the food industry because they reportedly provide many beneficial health effects. These effects include the regulation of intestinal microbial homeostasis (i.e., bacterial balance within the intestines), inhibition of pathogens and pathogenic bacteria that colonize and/or infect the gut mucosa. Other effects are modulation of local and systemic immune responses, production of vitamins, bioconversion of a number of dietary compounds into bioactive molecules, and repression of procarcinogenic enzymatic activities. *Bifidobacterium spp.*, for example, is known to discourage the growth of Gram-negative pathogens in infants. This apparently is because when mother's milk, which has high lactose content and a relatively lower buffering capacity with regard to acidity, is fermented by lactic acid bacteria (including *bifidobacteria*) in the infant's GI tract, the pH may drop into the acidic range. This drop in pH reduces the growth potential of Gram-negative bacteria.

Pathogenic ("Bad") Gram-positive bacteria

Streptococci are spherical bacteria that occur as chains with some streptococcal species being aerobic and others are anaerobic. In addition, certain species (i.e. alpha-hemolytic species) partly destroy red blood cells in blood agar culture media whereas others (termed beta-hemolytic) completely destroy the blood cells. *Streptococcal* species that do not destroy blood cells are referred to as gamma-hemolytic.

Although there are harmless streptococcal species involved in the production of yogurt, buttermilk and cheese, others are decidedly pathogenic. These include *Streptococcus pneumoniae,* the cause of secondary bacterial pneumonias, and *Streptococcus pyogenes,* causative agent of "strep throat".

Staphylococci occur in clusters and are normally present on the skin and in mucous membranes. Certain species of staphylococci are involved in skin pathologies such as boils, abscesses and carbuncles, notably when they produce coagulase, the enzyme that causes blood clotting. *Staphylococcus aureus* is involved in such pathologies as food poisoning, toxic shock syndrome, pneumonia and staphylococcal meningitis.

Bacillus and *Clostridium* species are rod-shaped bacteria that produce highly resistant spores which are found in the soil, air and within the body. Most species of *Bacillus* grow aerobically, and the deadliest species is *Bacillus anthracis,* the cause of anthrax. In contrast, *Clostridium* species grow anaerobically, and different species cause such pathological conditions as tetanus, botulism and gas gangrene. Interestingly, several *Bacillus* and *Clostridium* species have industrial applications, with certain *Clostridium* species being used to produce various chemicals, e.g. butyl alcohol or butanol, while *Bacillus thuringiensis* is used in insecticides against a variety of caterpillars.

Actinomyces species are Gram-positive rods that are anaerobic, with one species, *A. bovis,* causing the infection known as "lumpy jaw" that occurs in humans and cattle. Although *Actinomyces bovis* is a bacterium that is found normally in the mouths of healthy humans and animals, lumpy jaw is the result of an infection of the jawbone due to the bacteria entering small wounds in the mouth such as those caused by tooth eruption (teeth pushing through the gums) or coarse foodstuffs.

Aerobic and Anaerobic Bacteria

Bacteria are classified into two groups - aerobic and anaerobic - based on their requirement of oxygen. Anaerobic bacteria (anaerobes) are able to survive without the presence of oxygen whereas aerobic bacteria (aerobes) grow and multiply only in the presence of oxygen.

Anaerobic bacteria

There are three types of anaerobic bacteria. These are *obligate anaerobes* which cannot survive in the presence of oxygen, *aerotolerant anaerobes* which do not use oxygen for growth but can tolerate its presence, and *facultative anaerobes*, that can grow without oxygen but can use oxygen if it is present. Some anaerobic bacteria are pathogenic and can cause sinus infections, colds, fevers, ear infections and sexually transmitted diseases like syphilis, gonorrhea and chlamydia,. Anaerobic bacterial infections can be difficult to treat and often require extended antibiotic treatment for recalcitrant infections.

E. coli (Escherichia coli) is a common facultative (i.e. can live with or without oxygen) anaerobe present in the intestinal tract of human beings, mammals and birds but which can cause acute respiratory problems, diarrhea and urinary tract infections. One specific type of *E. coli (E. coli* 0157:H7) is very toxic and was identified only after an outbreak of food poisoning in the 1980s caused by consumption of undercooked beef in contaminated hamburgers.

Bacteroides is a genus of aerotolerant anaerobes that can infect various parts of the human body such as the peritoneal cavity and the female urogenital tract. However, some species of *Bacteroides* are beneficial to human beings.

Clostridium is a genus of rod-shaped obligate (i.e. cannot survive in the presence of oxygen) anaerobes with three main species. *C. botulinum* is found in improperly handled and/or contaminated meats and produces the extremely deadly toxin, botulinum. *C. tetani*, is found as a parasite in the gastrointestinal tract of animals as well as spores in soil; it produces a toxin called tetanospasmin, which causes tetanus. *C. perfringens* is found in dead and decaying vegetation, marine sediments and in the human intestinal tract; it causes such infections as food poisoning, gas gangrene and tissue necrosis.

Staphylococcus is a genus of facultative anaerobes that are found on the mucous membranes and human skin. One species, *Staphylococcus aureus* (*S. aureus*), can cause ordinary skin infections like boils and acne as well as potentially fatal infections like meningitis, pneumonia and toxic shock syndrome.

<u>Aerobic bacteria (aerobes)</u>

Obligate aerobic bacteria require oxygen for cellular respiration, that is, they need oxygen to survive, grow and reproduce although, as mentioned above, facultative bacteria (such as *E. coli and Staphylococcus spp.*) can behave both aerobically and anaerobically, depending on the prevailing conditions. There are also microaerophilic bacteria which require oxygen for their survival but only at very low concentrations. An example of a microaerophilic bacterium is *Helicobacter pylori (H. pylori),* which is present in patients with chronic gastritis and gastric ulcers, and is linked to the development of stomach cancer. However, over 80 percent of individuals infected with the bacterium are asymptomatic and *H. pylori* may play an important role in the natural stomach ecology.

The major roles of aerobic bacteria are in the recycling of nutrients, decomposing waste products and assisting in absorption of nutrients by plants. In fact, a wide variety of aerobes are known.

The genus *Bacillus* encompasses both obligate and facultative aerobes which range from the soil-dwelling *B. subtilis* to *B. anthracis* which causes anthrax. A variety of *Bacillus* species are used commercially in genetic research as well as in enzyme production.

Mycobacterium tuberculosis is a rod-shaped, obligate aerobe that causes tuberculosis by infesting the lungs of humans and mammals.

The genus *Nocardia* is a rod-shaped, Gram-positive bacterium with over 80 species, some of which are pathogenic and others are benign or non-pathogenic. *Nocardia* is normally present within the oral cavity, predominantly within the periodontal tissues, but it can cause nocardiosis which may affect only the lungs or the whole body.

Lactobacillus is not a true aerobic bacterium but is included in the category of facultative aerobes and *Lactobacillus spp.* are important in the fermentation of foodstuffs (e.g. production of yoghurt and cheese). This bacterium occurs routinely in the oral cavity and intestines, and some *Lactobacillus* species are beneficial to health, being classified as probiotic flora.

In addition to the strains discussed above, aerobic bacteria genera also include pathogenic species like *Pseudomonas, Staphylococcus* (facultative) and *Enterobacteriacae* spp. (facultative).

Good and Bad Bacteria

After the reader has labored through this chapter with its many classifications of bacteria and the incredible number of bacterial genera that inhabit the human body, it is understandable and probably a relief that the terms "good" and "bad" are so popular and in common use. A bacterium is "good" if it actually contributes to the health of its human (or animal) host or at least is non-pathogenic. On the other hand, a bacterium is "bad" if it is pathogenic or can interfere with the proper function of "good" bacteria. An example of the latter is when proliferation of "bad" bacteria displaces good bacteria from the oral or gut mucosa.

Antibiotics

As noted above, there are vast numbers of pathogenic bacteria which cause disease although the body is programmed to destroy invasive bacteria through the immune system. In situations where the immune system is compromised or cannot otherwise deal with bacterial infections, these pathogens customarily are dealt with by antimicrobials such as antibiotics. The latter either can kill bacteria (bactericidal action) or slow their growth by inhibition of multiplication (bacteriostatic action) so that they enhance the immune system's ability to deal with pathogens.

The first antibiotic was penicillin, discovered in 1928 by Sir Alexander Fleming, and it ushered in the antibiotic era. Medicine changed forever in the early 1950's, when large scale production of penicillin became possible. The term "antibiotic" originally was applied only to antimicrobials derived from living organisms such as molds, yeasts or other microorganisms. In contrast, "chemotherapeutic agents" are purely synthetic in origin although they have bacteriostatic or bactericidal activity against pathogenic microorganisms.

Nowadays, the term "antibiotic" is applied to all antimicrobials and includes naturally-derived, semi-synthetic and wholly synthetic therapeutics. Conventional antibiotics, however, are not effective in nonbacterial infections (e.g. those of viral or fungal origin) and individual antibiotics vary widely in their effectiveness on different species of bacteria.

Antibiotics typically are classified on the basis of target specificity. Narrow-spectrum antibiotics target particular types of microorganisms, e.g. gram-negative or gram-positive bacteria, whereas broad-spectrum antibiotics can affect a wider range of bacteria.

The effectiveness of an individual antibiotic varies with the location of the infection, its ability to reach the infection site and upon the ability of the bacteria to resist or inactivate the antibiotic. Whereas antibiotics are considered to be relatively harmless to the host, hence their use in treating infections, they often have an adverse effect on indigenous bacteria, particularly within the gut.

It has been found over the latter part of the 20th century and the early years of the 21st Century that there has been a diminution in the clinical effectiveness of antibiotics. There are various causes of this problem, including overuse and inappropriate use of antibiotics as well as mutations within many species of bacteria, so that some bacteria are resistant to all antibiotics. The prevalence of antibiotic resistance is rising, with some 60% of nosocomial (hospital acquired) infections now being antibiotic-resistant.

One approach to this problem has been the greater use of probiotics, both in the private sector as well as in clinical practice. In fact, both the Food and Agriculture Organization of the United Nations (FAO) and the World Health Organization (WHO) state that there is adequate scientific evidence of the potential for probiotic foods to provide health benefits.

3 PREBIOTICS

Chapters 1 and 2 indicated that the small and large intestines contain multiple species of microorganisms (bacteria). It was also stated that in the healthy body, the normal microflora comprises a balance in the numbers of beneficial and potentially harmful bacteria. Two bacterial species, Lactobacillus and Streptococcus, predominate in the small intestine whereas four species, *Bifidobacterium, Bacteroides, Eubacterium*, and *Peptostreptococcus*, are dominant in the colon or large intestine.

Unfortunately the delicate balance in the numbers and types of intestinal bacteria that should exist in healthy people can be disrupted by several factors, including poor diet, natural aging, stress and antibiotic therapy. An elevated intestinal pH (i.e. a more alkaline environment), for example, can cause a preponderance of "bad" bacteria. A bacterial imbalance that results in the preponderance or overgrowth of bad bacteria and yeast within the gut is known as intestinal dyspepsia.

The Digestive Process

The microbial flora in the gut digests foodstuffs by fermentation but the fermentation products differ with the foodstuffs being digested. In particular, fermentation products of carbohydrates differ from those of proteins, and these differences affect conditions within the gut.

Bacterial fermentation of carbohydrates (dietary fiber and compound sugars) yields short chain fatty acids, lactate, alcohols and aldehydes, the net result being an acidic environment in the gut. Carbohydrate fermentation also produces carbon dioxide (CO_2) and hydrogen (H_2), these gases subsequently interacting to form methane (CH_4) which eventually is passed as flatus, Figure 3.1.

Figure 3.1 *Bacterial fermentation of carbohydrates by intestinal microflora.*

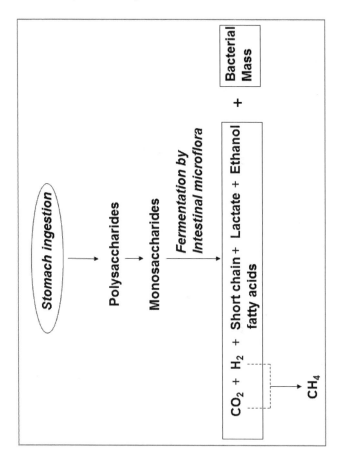

In contrast to carbohydrates, microbial fermentation of proteins produces branched chain fatty acids, amine compounds, H_2S (hydrogen sulfide), ammonia (NH_3), phenols, cresols and indoles, Figure 3.2.

Again, in contrast to carbohydrates, protein fermentation causes a rise in the intestinal pH, principally due to the generation of ammonia. It is noteworthy that several intestinal diseases, including irritable bowel syndrome and Crohn's disease, are associated with a high intestinal pH.

Thus differences in foodstuffs, i.e., the dietary intake, cause changes in the body's metabolism, with a greater carbohydrate intake being associated with a decrease in intestinal pH. Further, the gasses produced during fermentation increase the volume and reduce the transit time of the digested foodstuff in the intestine, thereby decreasing constipation.

Figure 3.2 *Bacterial fermentation of proteins by intestinal microflora*

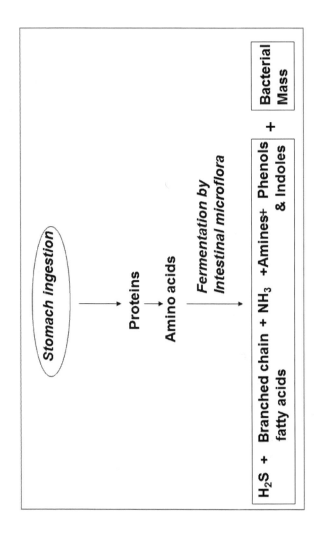

Clearly, parental admonitions to "eat your vegetables because they are good for you" have a sound scientific basis. In addition, many carbohydrates increase the water content of the intestine while the acids produced during fermentation increase intestinal motility. It is thought that the volatile fatty acids produced by fermentation both lower the pH of the colonic contents and provide protection for the colonic mucosa, thereby reducing the risk of colon cancer.

It should be added that some of these fermentation products enter into respiration which produces energy for the intestinal bacteria. The bacteria may also use this energy and the fermentation end-products for biosynthesis, which results in increased bacterial numbers.

Fruits, Vegetables and Gastric Health

One of the first physicians to explore the beneficial effects of starchless fruits and green leafy vegetables was Arnold Ehret (1866–1922), considered the "father" of naturopathic medicine. In his book, the *Mucusless Diet Healing System,* Ehret claimed that a diet of raw and cooked fruits and vegetables reduced/prevented mucus formation. He believed that these foodstuffs and a regimen of long- and short-term fasting provided effective colonic irrigation.

These insights were the result of Ehret contracting Bright's disease (a kidney disease) at the age of 31. After being told that he was incurable by the numerous physicians he consulted, Ehret adopted a vegetarian diet which he claimed cured his condition and this led him to explore natural healing and holistic medicine. In particular, he strongly advocated vegetarianism for cleansing and repairing the body due to the effects of poor nutrition and over-eating.

Following this change in diet, Ehret and fellow physician Bernard Jensen performed a number of autopsies. They found that 90 - 95% of the autopsied patients had clogged colons and the vast majority of these patients had suffered from chronic constipation.

This pioneering work of Ehret, and the findings of subsequent researchers, led to studies of the effects of fibrous foods on health.

The Nature of Prebiotics

Prebiotics are foodstuffs high in fiber which are not digested by the enzymes and acids in the stomach and pass virtually intact into the colon. Because these fibers are not digested in the upper gastrointestinal tract, they have minimal caloric value, i.e., they appear to have no nutritional effect, and they do not increase serum glucose or stimulate insulin secretion. However, once the fibers enter the colon, they are digested by the colonic microflora and produce short chain fatty acids.

The concept of prebiotics was first introduced in a scientific paper written by G. R. Gibson and M. B. Roberfroid, two scientists working at the Medical Research Council Dunn Nutrition Centre in Cambridge, England. This paper, entitled "Dietary modulation of the human colonic microbiota: introducing the concept of prebiotics", was published in the Journal of Nutrition in 1995 (see Bibliography) and was a landmark contribution to the scientific literature on nutrition.

Prebiotics were first defined as functional foods that were non-digestible but which stimulated the growth or activity of bacteria in the digestive system that were beneficial to the health of the body. This definition was later revised by Roberfroid in 2007 who defined a prebiotic as a selectively fermented ingredient that allows specific changes in both the composition and/or activity of the gastrointestinal microflora. As a result, a prebiotic will be beneficial to the well-being and health of the host.

Typically, prebiotics are carbohydrates (such as *oligosaccharides*), but non-carbohydrates were not precluded in the original definition of prebiotics. Only two fructooligosaccharides, namely oligofructose and inulin, fully satisfy Roberfroid's revised definition. Although other functional foodstuffs may be described as "prebiotic", it is increasingly common to refer to these other substances as "possible prebiotics", "likely prebiotics" or "having prebiotic activity".

Dietary Sources of Prebiotics

The most ubiquitous prebiotics are classed as soluble fibers, and many types of dietary fiber have prebiotic effects. The traditional dietary sources of prebiotic fibers, in alphabetical order, are indicated in Table 3.1.

Table 3.1 *Principal sources of inulin and dietary prebiotics*

Agave	Dandelions	Onions
Artichoke	Endives	Rye
Asparagus	Garlic	Soybeans
Bananas	Leeks	Wheat
Barley	Oats	Wild yam
Chicory		

While many components of dietary fiber such as digestion-resistant starch and non-starch polysaccharides provide substrates for fermentation by colonic bacteria, only fructooligosaccharides truly meet the qualifying criteria to be classified as prebiotics.

Fructooligosaccharides

Fructooligosaccharides are short- and medium-length chains of beta-D fructans, fructans being discussed next. Short-chain fructooligosaccharides are known as oligofructose whereas medium chain length fructooligosaccharides are known as inulin. The most studied prebiotic fibers are inulin and oligofructose, the latter being a subgroup of inulin. Inulin and oligofructose are plant storage carbohydrates found in over 36,000 plants worldwide.

Some oligosaccharides that occur naturally in breast milk are believed to be important in the development of a healthy immune system in infants. However, these compounds are not considered prebiotics, as they do not act through the intestinal microflora. Nevertheless, a recent study showed that breastfed babies and babies fed on prebiotic infant formula had a lower prevalence of atopic dermatitis than babies fed a normal formula. This finding suggests that prebiotics may have a beneficial effect on the development of the immune system.

The average U.S. diet provides 1–4 g of inulin and oligofructose per day (g/d) while the European diet averages 3–10 g/d; the difference arising from dietary and taste preferences. These dietary differences may be the source of differences in the gastric health of Americans and Europeans. Greater differences may exist between diets in other cultures.

Regardless of the average daily intake of dietary prebiotics, a case can be made for prebiotics supplementation. Much of the inulin and oligofructose commercially available is synthesized from sucrose or extracted from chicory roots which contain 15–20% inulin and 5–

10% oligofructose. Another widely used source of inulin is extracts of Jerusalem artichokes.

Commercially available ingredients include Raftilose (inulin hydrolysate) and Raftiline (inulin). Many commercial grades of inulin have a neutral flavor and are used to improve the texture, stability and palatability of low fat foods.

In contrast, oligofructose has a sweet flavor and is highly soluble. Consequently, it is often used to fortify foods with fiber to improve flavor, palatability and texture of reduced-fat foods.

Prebiotic oligosaccharides increasingly are added to commercially-produced foods for their perceived health benefits. Such additives include polydextrose and some oligosaccharides, notably fructo-, xylo- and galactooligosaccharides. Monosaccharides such as tagatose are also added to human foodstuffs as prebiotics while certain mannooligosaccharides are likewise added to pet foodstuffs.

Fructans

A fructan is a polymer of fructose (or sugar) molecules. Fructans with a short chain length are known as fructooligosaccharides, whereas longer chain fructans are termed inulins. Fructans occur in foods such as agave, artichokes, asparagus, leeks, garlic, onions (including spring onions) and wheat, Table 3.1. The fructan contents of various foods are given in Table 3.2.

Table 3.2 *Fructan content of various foods*

Foodstuff	Fructan content (%)
Artichoke, Jerusalem	16 - 20
Artichoke, Globe	2 - 7
Asparagus	1 - 4
Chocolate	9
Garlic	17
Onion	1 - 10
Pasta	1- 4
Rye (bran)	7
Wheat flour	1- 4
White bread	1 - 3

Fructose, or fruit sugar, is a simple monosaccharide found in many plants that was discovered by the French chemist Augustin-Pierre Dubrunfaut in 1847. Along with glucose and galactose, fructose is one of the three dietary monosaccharides that are absorbed directly into the bloodstream during digestion.

Pure, dry fructose is a very sweet, white, odorless, crystalline solid and is the most water-soluble of all the sugars. Fructose is found in honey, tree and vine fruits, flowers, berries and most root vegetables. Fructose may be present in plants as the monosaccharide and/or as a component of sucrose. The latter is a disaccharide with a molecule of glucose and a molecule of fructose bonded together with a glycosidic linkage. Most modern fruits and vegetables have been bred to have much higher sugar content than the wild plants from which they descended.

Functions of Prebiotics

It has long been recognized that the microbiota of the human gut can have a major impact on host health. This awareness led to attempts to manipulate the composition of the gut flora by increasing levels of such beneficial bacterial species as *Bifidobacterium* and *Lactobacillus.* Microbial food supplements also have been used to change the composition of colonic microbiota. These supplements, claimed to beneficially affect the host through their effect on intestinal microbial balance, are known as Probiotics (Chapter 4).

However, it has been argued that changes in microbial balance from exogenous bacteria may be transient and their effectiveness limited. Probiotic supplements, to be effective, must contain significant numbers of living microorganisms. In particular, if the ingested bacteria are to have any effect in the colon, they must survive exposure to the acids and digestive enzymes in the stomach and small intestine.

Consequently, it has been suggested that only limited numbers of probiotic bacteria survive passage through the stomach and small intestine to the colon.

As previously stated, prebiotics are non-digestible food ingredients that selectively stimulate the growth and/or activity of one or a limited number of bacteria in the colon. In other words, they improve host health *by* boosting the numbers of beneficial bacteria and/or increase carbohydrate metabolism. This conclusion is based on the assumption *that it is beneficial to health* to increase carbohydrate fermentation and to suppress protein fermentation in the intestine. In effect, ingestion of prebiotics will modulate the endogenous colonic microbiota by increasing the levels of specific bacteria, thereby changing the composition of the microbiota.

Gibson and Roberfroid, the originators of the prebiotic concept, also suggested that fermentation products of prebiotics modulate lipid metabolism. However, such a change in metabolic activity does not necessarily correlate with an increase in the numbers of the possible beneficial bacterial groups.

The definition of a prebiotic does not specify any particular bacterial group although it is generally assumed that the number and/or activity of bifidobacteria and lactic acid bacteria (LABs) are affected. The bifidobacteria and the LABs are important because they appear to improve digestion and enhance mineral absorption. They are also thought to enhance the effectiveness and intrinsic strength of the immune system.

Agents that stimulate bifidobacteria are considered bifidogenic factors. However, not all prebiotics are bifidogenic since they may stimulate other (beneficial) bacteria in the intestinal flora. On the other hand, many non-digestible oligosaccharides are not prebiotic and, in fact, may be inert or even exert harmful effects. A more recent development has been the concept of symbiosis; namely combining prebiotics and probiotics into a single product that has a health-enhancing function. The underlying concept is that the prebiotic is beneficial to flora in the small intestine and the probiotic benefits the flora in the large intestine. This is actually a misunderstanding of the role and actions of prebiotics and probiotics. Probiotics, as discussed in Chapter 4, have no effect in the large intestine whereas prebiotics, which function only in the large intestine, are unlikely to stimulate the action of probiotics in the small intestine.

The mechanism whereby prebiotics have a beneficial or stimulatory influence on the immune system is probably a secondary effect arising from stimulation and support of the flora within the colon. Since some 80% of the body's immune cells are within the colon, stimulation of the colonic flora by prebiotics will have a beneficial effect on the overall immune system.

Effects of Prebiotics

Regardless of the actual mechanism of action, prebiotics act on the flora in the large intestine and have a variety of beneficial effects. These include improved absorption of calcium and other minerals and enhanced immune system effectiveness, Table 3.3.

Table 3.3 *Beneficial effects of prebiotics.*

Restoration of intestinal bacterial balance
Reduction of intestinal pH
Improved bowel regularity
Increased *Bifidobacterium* and *Lactobacillus* levels
Increased absorption of calcium and magnesium
Reduction in serum cholesterol levels
Stabilized microflora in infants
Stimulation of the immune system
Reduced risk of colorectal cancer
Improved intestinal flora in infants
Improved glycemic and blood sugar control
Improved control of appetite and weight
Moderated flatus odor
Reduced gut levels of *Clostridium* and *Bacteroides*

Based upon widely reported research findings, gastroenterologists suggest that prebiotics may help treat a number of conditions, Table 3.4.

Table 3.4 *Prebiotics in gastroenterology*

Colon cancer
Colon gas and flatulence
Colon polyps
Crohn's disease
Dietary therapy for colon pathology
Diverticulosis
Irritable bowel syndrome
Ulcerative colitis

The Food and Drug Administration (FDA) prohibits claims by the dietary supplement industry that their products can prevent, cure or mitigate any disease. Thus, although no specific claims can be made regarding the effectiveness of prebiotics (or probiotics), there is increasing evidence that both prebiotics and probiotics can have markedly beneficial effects on the body.

Constipation

Possibly, the most common application of prebiotics and probiotics is in the relief of constipation. Constipation, also known as costiveness as well as by the medical terms of dyschezia and dyssynergic defecation, is a condition in which bowel movements are infrequent and it is a common cause of painful defecation. It is quite common, with a general prevalence of between 2 to 30% although, as noted by Ehret and Jensen, 90 - 95% of autopsied patients had clogged colons and the vast majority of these presumably older patients had suffered from chronic constipation.

Constipation is a symptom rather than a disease *per se*, and has many different causes although two types predominate. The first, obstructed defecation, appears to affect about 50% of patients referred to hospital for treatment and appears have both mechanical and functional causes. The other cause of constipation is slow transit of digested foodstuffs through the colon or hypomotility. Many things contribute to hypomotility, including diet, hormones, medications and heavy metal toxicity.

Slow intestinal passage or transit of digested foodstuffs, i.e. one cause of constipation *is relieved by* dietary fiber, known as *prebiotics.* Most prebiotics are carbohydrates that are fermented in the large intestine and the gases produced during fermentation increase the volume and reduce the transit time of the fecal material in the large intestine. Prebiotics also increase the water content and lower the pH in the intestine, both effects enhancing gut motility, reduce transit time, and help relieve constipation.

Other Effects of Prebiotics

It is possible that the observed effects of prebiotics may be due to stimulation of colonic bacteria and a possible change in metabolism and increased dietary carbohydrates. The prebiotic-induced metabolism change, i.e. more carbohydrate and less protein fermentation, lowers the intestinal pH and this may reduce (but not cure) the symptoms of Crohn's disease and irritable bowel syndrome.

The propensity of prebiotics to stimulate bacteria appears to restore the intestinal bacterial balance following such insults as antibiotics, stress, therapeutic drugs, and diarrhea. This may be due to direct stimulation of certain groups of bacteria that grow on the prebiotics or by indirect stimulation which may induce the proliferation of other bacteria. In this context, it is known that many oral pathogens may destabilize the normal microflora of young children. Several studies have shown that commercial oligosaccharides can stabilize pediatric microflora by changing the microflora and reducing the pH (i.e., increasing the acidity).

It has been suggested that certain oligosaccharides can benefit blood cholesterol levels and reduce the risk of colorectal cancer although neither effect has been proven in clinical studies. There are indications that protein fermentation products (by causing a more basic or higher pH) may increase the risk of colorectal cancer, the latter may be reduced through increased carbohydrate fermentation, which lowers the pH to more acidic levels.

Studies on the effect of the intestinal microflora on the immune system have not clearly demonstrated a beneficial effect for prebiotics. However, by changing the intestinal flora, prebiotics may influence the immune system.

High Fiber Diets

The principal function of the colon is to complete the digestion process by removing excess water from food waste entering from the small intestine. If the waste matter transits the intestines too quickly, insufficient water is absorbed, causing watery stools and diarrhea. When transit of waste is too slow, too much water is absorbed, causing hard stools and constipation.

Modern physicians, gastroenterologists and dieticians advocate high fiber diets to alleviate these problems; echoing the admonitions of Ehret early in the 20th century. Dietary fiber (also called roughage or bulk) is the indigestible part of plant cell walls responsible for the structure of the plant. It includes cellulose, hemicellulose, polysaccharides, pectins, gums, mucilages, and lignins, the majority of which are not digested by the body. This resistance to digestion affects both the normal functioning and disorders of the large intestine.

Dietary fiber promotes the wavelike contractions (peristalsis) that move food through the intestines and facilitate the passage of fecal waste. Fibrous substances also absorb many times their weight in water, resulting in softer, bulkier stools which pass through the bowel more easily and quickly. This elimination-easing action of fibrous material may avoid, halt and even reverse some digestive tract disorders. Not only do softer, larger stools help prevent constipation, straining, and the development of hemorrhoids, they reduce pressure within the colon. The latter is an important factor in the treatment of irritable bowel syndrome (IBS) as well as treating ulcerative bowel syndrome and diverticulosis. The lower prevalence of digestive tract diseases in rural populations compared to urban dwellers is related to the high-fiber nature of their diet. It is also possible a faster rate of fecal waste elimination will facilitate expulsion of harmful substances before they can cause problems.

Other research suggests that dietary fiber and prebiotics may be important in treating diabetes, elevated cholesterol, colon polyps, and cancer of the colon although the findings are not definitive. Soluble fibers such as psyllium mucilloid not only regulate bowel function but also reduce cholesterol, possibly by binding with it in bile and eliminating it in the stool. Table 3.5 indicates common foodstuffs high in dietary fiber.

Table 3.5 *High dietary fiber foodstuffs*

Whole grain foods* (e.g. bran cereals)
Whole wheat bread*
Fresh fruit (including the skin and pulp)
Dried or stewed fruits (raisins, prunes, apricots)
Root vegetables (carrots, potatoes, turnips)
Raw or fresh vegetables (notably cabbage)

(oat bran and bread provide both insoluble and soluble fibers)*

Excessive intake of dietary fibers, however, can bind and reduce absorption of certain minerals such as calcium, copper, iron, magnesium, selenium and zinc. Long-term adaptation to high fiber intakes does occur, but the immediate addition of substantial quantities of fibers and prebiotics to the diet may result in a temporary increase in gas, bloating, or bowel movements.

Healthy diets require plentiful ingestion of fluids (water and fruit/vegetable juices). Slow and thorough eating of food will promote its breakdown by saliva and digestive juices in the stomach or the lower intestines.

Bibliography for Chapter 3

Coxam V; Current data with inulin-type fructans and calcium, targeting bone health in adults. J Nutr (2007) 137(11 Suppl): P-2527S.

Geier MS et al; Probiotics, prebiotics and synbiotics: a role in chemoprevention for colorectal cancer? Cancer Biol Ther (2006) 5(10): 1265-9

Gibson GR, Roberfroid MB. Dietary modulation of the human colonic microbiota: introducing the concept of prebiotics. J Nutr. (1995) 125(6):1401-12.

Hedin C et al. Evidence for the use of probiotics and prebiotics in inflammatory bowel disease: a review of clinical trials. Proc Nutr Soc. (2007) 66(3): 307-15.

Katharina E. Scholz-Ahrens, JS. Inulin and oligofructose and mineral metabolism: the evidence from animal trials. J Nutr. (2007) 137: 2513S

Lomax AR, Calder PC. Prebiotics, immune function, infection and inflammation: a review of the evidence. Institute of Human Nutrition, School of Medicine, University of Southampton, Tremona Road, Southampton, UK

Macfarlane S et al; Prebiotics in the gastrointestinal tract. Aliment Pharmacol Ther. (2006) 24(5): 701-14.

Marcel Roberfroid; Prebiotics: the concept revisited. J Nutr. 2007; 137: 830S

Roberfroid MB. Prebiotics: The concept revisited. J Nutr. (2007) 137: 830S

Seifert S, Watzl B. Inulin and Oligofructose: Review of experimental data on immune modulation. J Nutr. (2007) 137: 2563S.

4 PROBIOTICS

An important facet of 21st Century culture is that good mental and physical health depends upon a balanced, nutritious diet, daily exercise, a stress-free environment and strong interpersonal relationships. These precepts are built, at least in part, on the work of a Russian physician, Eli Metchnikoff. In particular, he examined the lifestyles of Bulgarian people in the early years of the 20th Century because of anecdotal reports that these Eastern Europeans had virtually no serious medical problems. Metchnikoff also noted that these Bulgarian people enjoyed tremendous vitality and unusually long lives, many living for 100 years or more.

Metchnikoff attributed this extraordinary longevity and outstanding health, compared to that of the rest of the world, to dietary differences. Of particular interest was the fact that the Bulgarian people he studied consumed large amounts of natural yoghurt. Examination of this natural yoghurt showed that it was cultured by two microorganisms which he isolated and identified, namely *Lactobacillus bulgaricus* and *Streptococcus thermophilus.* These findings were supported by the long-held tradition of physicians in the Near- and Middle-East of treating digestive (gastrointestinal) disorders, liver problems and poor appetite with soured milk.

Metchnikoff believed that absorption of toxins generated and released by bacteria within the biosystem shortened the human life span. It was his contention, supported by the venerable medical traditions of Mesopotamia and the Levant, that the microorganisms in yoghurt slowed or reversed the adverse health effects of pathogens in the intestinal tract.

These theories on health and intestinal microbiology were largely ignored for many decades. There was a resurgence of interest in them, however, with the growing awareness by the medical profession and the public at large of the adverse health effects of professional and personal stress on individuals. Changes in attitude with regard to the GI tract were also prompted towards the end of the 20th Century by the realization that poor diet, sedentary lifestyles, widespread use of drugs and antibiotics and a variety of other environmental challenges could have a major, usually negative, impact on the intestinal microflora. This, in turn, led to the realization that any such changes in microflora would have a deleterious effect on gastrointestinal (GI) health and, presumably, affect the whole body.

It is now widely accepted that certain microorganisms, notably those derived from fermented milk products, are beneficial to the health and viability of the GI tract. In particular, microorganisms such as *L. bulgaricus* and *S. thermophilus* are now recognized as being able to provide support for a healthy indigenous intestinal flora and alleviate many digestive problems.

Probiotics and their Sources

The term *probiotics* derives from the Greek word *biotiks* or life. As defined by the World Health Organization (WHO) and the Food and Agricultural Organization of the United Nations (FAO), probiotics are living microorganisms which confer health benefits on the host when administered in adequate amounts. Currently, probiotics are accepted to be concentrated supplements of live microbial food that benefit the host. This health improvement stems from their effect on the intestinal microbial balance, the latter preventing or reversing the adverse effects of pathogenic bacteria on the body.

A plethora of probiotic formulations is now available from health food stores and internet sites. Increasingly, larger food manufacturers market yoghurts that also contain these "protective" bacteria. Although probiotic formulations and their bacterial counts differ with the manufacturer, most products contain one or more of the most commonly used bacteria, Table 5.1. It should be noted that a considerable number of probiotic bacterial species have been identified and each can comprise up to hundreds of separate strains. The genus Lactobacillus, for example, has 60 or so species and is the fermenting agent used to preserve and flavor food like sauerkraut and sausage.

Complicating the issue is the fact that each bacterial strain may have different health effects despite close relationships to each other so that the characteristics of probiotic bacteria can vary markedly. Bifidobacteria such as Lactospore® and *Lactobacillus sporogenes* (now known as *Bacillus coagulans*) are spore formers and produce lactic acid whereas *Saccharomyces boulandii* is a yeast culture.

Many species, notably *Lactobacillus acidophilus, Lactobacillus paracasei, Lactobacillus plantarum, Lactobacillus rhamnosus* and *Lactobacillus salivarius,* are common in the mucosa that extends from the mouth to the anus in humans. Of the species cited in Table 4.1, *L. paracasei* and *L. rhamnosus* are usually associated with fermented dairy products whereas *L. plantarum* occurs in fermented plant foods.

Many bacteria that occur naturally in the gut produce lactic acid and promote healthy GI microbial systems. The lactic acid metabolite from probiotic bacteria helps digest foods, improves the bioavailability of minerals and supports production of B vitamins within the body. This is important for lactose-intolerant individuals because the bacteria produce lactose-hydrolyzing enzymes, clearly benefiting the digestive health of the individual.

Table 4.1 *Widely used probiotic bacteria*

Lactobacillus acidophilus	Bifidobacterium bifidum
Lactobacillus bifidum	Bifidobacterium breve
Lactobacillus brevis	Bifidobacterium lactis
Lactobacillus bulgaricus	Bifidobacterium longum
Lactobacillus casei	Bifidus regularis
Lactobacillus gasseri	
Lactobacillus helveticus	Pediococcus acidilactici
Lactobacillus infantis	
Lactobacillus lactis	Saccharomyces boulandii
Lactobacillus longum	
Lactobacillus paracasei	Streptococcus salivarius
Lactobacillus plantarum	Streptococcus thermophilus
Lactobacillus rhamnosus	
Lactobacillus salivarius	
Lactobacillus sporogenes*	
(* Now Bacillus coagluans)	

There are many other probiotic functional foods that are not yoghurts. These include the lactic acid fermented oatmeal gruel consumed in Sweden, the Tanzanian beverage, Togwa, and the fermented milk drink, Kefir. Kefir has been consumed for hundreds of years in the Caucasus region because of the strongly-held belief that it helps maintain the strength of the stomach and immune system although the immune system obviously was unheard of when Kefir was first produced.

Many probiotic bacteria have high proteolytic activity, that is, they can cleave proteins, an action that facilitates their digestion and absorption by the body. This may account for their effectiveness in alleviating digestive problems, the primary use of probiotic supplements. However, there are indications that probiotics also provide other support to the physiology of the biosystem. Many probiotic bacteria have bacteriocins as metabolic by-products, bacteriocins possessing antibiotic-like behavior, a characteristic of obvious importance when pathogenic bacteria are present within the body.

Milk and milk derivatives

Milk is a complex mixture of fats, proteins and other compounds and is the first source of nourishment for the offspring of humans and animals. The nutritional value of milk has been recognized for thousands of years and, unsurprisingly, the majority of probiotics are based on lactic acid fermentation of milk as well as its constituents.

The sources of milk determines its composition with clear differences, e.g. in the lactose content, existing between human, bovine, goat and other types of milk. Nevertheless there is a certain commonality in that all milks contain approximately 5% lactose, 4% lipids, 0.7% mineral salts and 3.2% protein but the smaller differences define the character and source of this essential foodstuff. In particular, each type of milk contains a variety of proteins and complex sugars as well as a spectrum of bioactive agents, such as lactoferrin and lactoperoxidase. The latter is an enzyme secreted from various mucosal glands and which is a potent bactericidal agent. Because lactoperoxidase catalyzes the oxidation of many inorganic and organic substrates by hydrogen peroxide, this complex of the enzyme together with its inorganic ion substrates, hydrogen peroxide and oxidized products is known as the lactoperoxidase system. The latter is important to the innate immune system by killing bacteria in milk and mucosal secretions while having no effect on DNA and it is not mutagenic.

About 80% of the total protein content of milk is casein. Although casein itself has no physiological role in the body, casein-derived proteins are bioactive and are detectable in the stomach after ingestion of milk or yoghurt. Various casein-derived peptides are absorbed and detected in plasma, again indicating the physiological activity of milk-derived peptides.

In addition to its obvious nutritional value, milk's usefulness in preventing infection has been recognized for millennia. At one time, anti-infection activity was attributed largely to antibodies and immunoglobulins but while that perception has changed with progress in microbiology, recognition of milk's importance in systemic health has not. The impact of milk ingestion on pre-eruptive tooth mineralization and, later, its effects on dental decay was first advocated some 80 years ago. It is unsurprising, therefore, that milk and such derivatives as yoghurt and cheese have a major impact on systemic and oral health.

The previously mentioned lactoferrin, found in breast and bovine milk and mucosal secretions such as tears and saliva, has been shown to be highly effective against a broad range of microorganisms. The latter include gram-positive and gram-negative bacteria as well as yeasts such as *Candida albicans*. Interestingly, human colostrum (so-called "first milk" secreted immediately after childbirth) has the highest concentration of lactoferrin. Although lower levels of lactoferrin are found in breast milk (and in cow's milk), these findings support the beneficial effect of breast-feeding for babies. It is also worth mentioning that pepsin-mediated digestion of lactoferrin in gastric juices produces lactoferricin, a peptide with anti-microbial and anti-cancer properties.

The scientific literature indicates that infections caused by probiotics based on lactobacilli and bifidobacteria species are extremely rare. This absence of pathogenicity appears to extend across all age groups and even to immune-compromised individuals.

Physiological Effects of Probiotics

The improved health and stimulation of natural immunity against a variety of pathogens by probiotics, i.e. their physiological benefits, has been ascribed to their ability to competitively reduce the numbers of pathogenic bacteria within the biosystem. In particular, the probiotic bacteria become the dominant microbial species and, by reducing the pathogenic bacterial population, they provide protection against, and possibly cure, various diseases. This action is known as bacteriotherapy or bacterioprophylaxis but, more commonly, is called replacement therapy.

The basis of replacement therapy is the implantation of relatively innocuous "effector" bacteria within the normal microflora. Provided these effector bacteria can maintain a continuing presence within the normal microflora, they can prevent the colonization and proliferation of potentially disease-causing (pathogenic) bacteria in the target environment without disturbing the balance of the existing microbial ecosystem.

Replacement therapy has a long history. In 1877, over 135 years ago, Pasteur and Joubert proposed using an effector strain of bacteria to replace pathogens and control bacterial disease. Although the ready availability of antibiotics appeared to eliminate the clinical need for bacteriotherapy over the past 60 or so years, there has been reawakening of interest because of the short half-life (i.e., clinical usefulness) of most antimicrobials and growing problem of antibiotic-resistant bacteria.

Despite the effectiveness and long history of replacement therapy, microbial interference is not wholly understood. One conjecture is that the effector bacteria adhere to surfaces and compete more successfully for limited space and nutrients than the pathogens they displace. An alternative view is that effector bacteria have a greater capacity for reproduction and are more resistant than the displaced pathogens to non-specific antibacterial agents such as peroxides and acids. A third possibility (amongst many others) is that effector bacteria are inherently more resistant to therapeutic agents administered to act on relatively similar bacteria. It should be noted in this context that bacteriophages, bacteriocins and bacteriocin-like inhibitory substances (BLIS) can act as natural antibiotics and control the growth of bacterial pathogens. This treatment regimen has used for 100 years or more in France, Russia and Eastern Europe.

Probiotics and GI health

It is often argued that poor nutrition (i.e. an unbalanced diet) and ingestion of antibiotics, antacids, alcohol, etc., facilitates proliferation of "bad" bacteria which in turn results in a multiplicity of conditions. The qualitative and quantitative stability of the normal, indigenous microflora in healthy people limits invasion and overgrowth by pathogenic bacteria. The intrinsic stability of the indigenous microbiota, that is, the equilibrium between microbial species in normal microflora, inhibits modifications to its composition. This equilibrium between bacterial species, however, can be disrupted by nutritional, hormonal and/or physical changes as well as by chemical agents such as antibiotics and antacids. It is well-known that psychological stress, for example, affects bacterial balance within the digestive system. A result of the increasing pressures experienced in the 21st Century is that gastric ulcers, and their associated bacteria (*H. pylori*), are now relatively common afflictions.

Any significant reduction in the numbers of individual components of the bacterial population in the micro-environment can result in overgrowth by previously suppressed minority elements. The common symptoms associated with bacterial overgrowth are bloating, abdominal pain, increased flatulence and diarrhea. A complication of the increasingly common gastric bypass surgery treatment for obesity can be an alteration in gastrointestinal flora which can lead to bacterial overgrowth.

A new study of obese patients who underwent gastric bypass surgery at Stanford University Medical School has found that probiotic supplementation following gastric bypass surgery may prevent bacterial overgrowth. Compared to controls that did not receive probiotics, patients receiving probiotics had lower levels of bacterial overgrowth 6 months after surgery, had a greater weight loss and a

50% higher level of vitamin B-12 than the control group.

A study performed in France and published in July of 2009 in the *British Journal of Nutrition* investigated the effect of probiotics on women suffering from regular digestive problems rather than gastrointestinal diseases. One group received yogurt supplemented with probiotics and the other a non-fermented dairy product and both groups were followed for a month. It was found that improvements in gastrointestinal health (digestive symptoms and evaluations of digestive comfort) of women receiving the probiotic yogurt were significantly greater than for those in the placebo group. However, it was noted that the benefits from probiotic supplementation disappeared within a month after cessation of supplementation. This suggests that continued supplementation is necessary to maintain gastrointestinal well-being.

Several studies indicate that probiotics can help prevent and treat diarrhea, even in people on antibiotics. Antibiotic-related diarrhea is relatively common (i.e. a prevalence of 20-30%) with children, and many parents will stop antibiotic therapy or seek further medical treatment to alleviate the diarrhea. There is evidence that the antibiotic-rich kefir can treat or prevent antibiotic-induced diarrhea, and appears to be most effective with younger, sicker children. This may be the result of boosting the immune system, an action less necessary for healthier pediatric patients. Reports indicate the duration of episodes of acute watery diarrhea in children caused by rotavirus is decreased by several types of probiotics.

The widespread acceptance of the effectiveness of probiotics in maintaining the health of the gut is based upon recolonization of the intestinal microflora which protects the stomach lining. This in turn reduces the severity of acute diarrhea in children as well as preventing/treating antibiotic-associated diarrhea and inflammatory bowel disease. *Lactobacillus salivarius*, for example, is thought to be a potentially effective probiotic against *Helicobacter pylori*, a bacterium that causes chronic low-level inflammation ulcers and stomach cancer. However, other scientific work suggests that probiotic bacteria may not eliminate *Helicobacter pylori* (*H. pylori*).

Probiotics and Systemic Health

The majority of probiotics studies reported in the scientific literature have focused on the prevention and treatment of gastrointestinal disease and allergies (see later). There is, however, a growing number of claims that probiotics are effective against other conditions, Table 4.2.

In other words, the health effects of ingested probiotic micro-organisms are not confined to the intestines because many systemic health problems originate, at least in part, from adverse conditions within the colon. These include yeast-associated conditions, ulcers, dermatitis, acne, sinus problems, allergies, halitosis, colds, influenza and other problems involving the immune system. Headaches and anxiety/mood swings also have been ascribed to bacterial imbalance within the colon.

The wider health benefit claims are based on the presumption that by maintaining or improving the barrier function of the intestinal mucosa, probiotics may inhibit translocation of potential pathogens. This should prevent infections of the blood stream and the correlated adverse effects on other tissues and organs. However, as mentioned in elsewhere, changes in microbial balance arising from exogenous bacteria may be transient and of limited effectiveness. The effectiveness of probiotics in controlling yeast infections, for example, is debatable. In the overall context of probiotics and health, probiotics and other supplements commonly are consumed by healthy and health-conscious people. However, it is somewhat ironic that little is known about the effect of probiotics on the immune system of the healthy individual.

Table 4.2 *Common claims for benefits of probiotics therapy*

Alleviation of digestive disorders

Control of pathogenic bacteria

Control of yeasts

Diminished gas, bloating and abdominal pain

Diminished irritable bowel syndrome

Enhanced metabolization of B vitamins

Immune system enhancement

Improve immune function

Improved absorption of calcium and magnesium

Improved digestion

Prevention and treatment of diarrhea

Prevention and treatment of pediatric respiratory infections

Prevention of recurrence of superficial bladder cancer

Relief of constipation and diarrhea

Reduction in some allergic reactions

Restoration of natural microflora balance after stress, antibiotic therapy, alcohol use and chemotherapy.

Probiotics and the Immune System

The supporting data for the claims of apocryphal reports of the action of probiotics in alleviating and possibly curing the symptoms and conditions indicated in Table 4.2 are not always clear-cut or scientifically validated. On the other hand, some 80% of the body's immune cells are located within the gut so that if probiotics do ensure a healthy balance of the intestinal microflora, there is a logical basis for claims regarding their beneficial effects upon the immune system.

It does appear that probiotics may modulate immune responses via the gut's mucosal immune system. In particular, probiotics appear to have an anti-inflammatory action. This was shown by a probiotics-related decrease in serum CRP (C-Reactive Protein), the latter being produced in the liver during episodes of acute inflammation or infection. Probiotics also appear to reduce bacteria-induced production of pro-inflammatory cytokines. These findings suggest that probiotics may be helpful for patients suffering from various types of inflammatory or autoimmune diseases.

Research studies reported from China and the United States indicate that the *Lactobacillus species* of probiotics stimulate the immune system. Children suffering from colds and influenza showed a 73% reduction in the occurrence of fevers, a 59% reduction in runny noses and a 62% drop in the prevalence of coughing when they received probiotics compared to controls.

Allergic reactions are linked to the immune system and probiotics were found to be somewhat beneficial for young children born to pregnant women who were at high risk of developing allergies. and symptoms also appear to be alleviated by probiotics, again suggesting beneficial effects on the immune system. Research findings indicate that infants who received perinatal probiotics (i.e. the mothers took probiotics during the last month of pregnancy) appeared to be free of allergies up to the age of 2 years. However, this protective effect was not found after the children reached the age of 5. It was also noted that babies born by cesarean section had a lower prevalence of allergies when they were exposed to perinatal probiotics compared to controls.

Despite these favorable reports on the efficacy of probiotics, it has to be stated that further research is necessary before the therapeutic claims made for probiotic ingestion are completely validated.

Probiotics and Diet

The many and varied claims by probiotic therapy advocates appear to be in accord with the bacteriotherapy theory of Pasteur and Joubert. However, the vast majority of these interested parties appear to neglect or disregard the role of prebiotics and dietary fiber on intestinal health. This apparent omission deviates from the teachings of Arnold Ehret, the man considered to be the father of naturopathic medicine and, apparently, the clinical use of probiotics. Since bacteria require a substrate to colonize and from which base they are able to proliferate, it is reasonable to suggest that prebiotics or at least a high fiber diet should be consumed in addition to probiotics, although not necessarily at the same time.

It is claimed that probiotics, by stimulating the colonization and proliferation of "good" bacteria, alleviate the above pathologic conditions. However, in order to maximize the benefits of probiotic therapy, probiotics manufacturers maintain that certain guidelines, Table 4.3, must be followed.

Table 4.3 *Recommendations for probiotic therapy*

Avoid heat-applied enteric-coated capsules
Avoid use of antibiotics and antacids
Take sufficiently high numbers of bacteria (5 billion or more)
Use multi-strain probiotics

These guidelines appear to be reasonable, particularly avoiding heat-applied enteric coated probiotic capsules and antacids. Probiotics are living organisms, their viability is determined by storage conditions, time elapsed between packaging and consumption, and temperature variations to which these products are subjected. An additional consideration with regard to probiotics is that the product should be packaged such that it is protected from light, air, elevated temperatures and moisture, all of which can adversely affect if not kill the probiotic bacteria.

Probiotic supplements must contain very large numbers of living microorganisms and in order to be effective, they must resist the acids and digestive enzymes in the stomach and small intestine in order to survive these assaults and still be viable once they reach the colon. In fact, some authorities suggest that the survival of exogenous bacteria (i.e. bacteria in probiotics) on passage through the stomach, large and small intestines to the colon may be limited. Enteric coatings and specialized encapsulation techniques, however, are claimed to preserve the viability of probiotic bacteria on passage through the small intestine to the colon. Another factor affecting the viability of probiotic bacteria is the consumption of antacids which, by elevating the intestinal pH, will tend to kill the bacteria.

The optimal number of bacteria to be taken on a daily basis is unknown but it appears that *more is better than less* to compensate for destruction of the ingested bacteria being lost on transit through the stomach and intestines. Current thinking appears to be that at least each gram of yoghurt or probiotic-containing drink must contain one million (10^6) of each type of probiotic bacterium for effectiveness.

The particular strains of probiotic bacteria that have the greatest effectiveness is not established and probably varies with the individual. Accordingly, most manufacturers formulate supplements containing up to 10-15 different strains, presumably because bacterial intestinal vary with the individual so that some of the bacteria will be more active than others.

To date, most studies of the health benefits of probiotics have focused on the *Lactobacillus* and *Bifidobacterium* strains, and these are the dominant species in most supplement formulations. Nevertheless, it is surprising that little attention has been paid to other lactic acid fermentation products. There appears to be little interest, for example, in the antimicrobial and anti-Candidal properties of lactoferricin.

Bibliography

Aiba Y, Suzuki N, et al. Lactic acid-mediated suppression of Helicobacter pylori by the oral administration of Lactobacillus salivarius as a probiotic in a gnotobiotic murine model. Am J Gastroenterol (1998) 93:2097-101.

Aimutis WR. Bioactive properties of milk proteins with particular focus on anticariogenesis J. Nutr (2004) 134:989S-995S.

Balansky, R. Inhibitory effects of freeze-dried milk fermented by selected *Lactobacillus bulgaricus* strains on carcinogenesis induced by 1,2-dimethylhydrazine in rats and by diethylnitrosamine in hamsters. *Cancer Letters (1999)* 147(1-2): 125-37.

Bengmark S. Pre-, pro- and symbiotics. Curr Opin Clin Nutr Metab Care (2001) 4: 571-579.

Bergman SA, von Fraunhofer JA. The plain person's guide to immunology. Am Dent Institute (2004) 86: 3-11.

Beshkova, D. Production of amino acids by yogurt bacteria. *Biotechnology Progress (1998) 14(6): 963-95.*

Bibel, DL. Bacterial interference, bacteriotherapy and bacterioprophylaxis. In: Bacterial interference (ed. R. Aly and H. R. Shinefield), CRC Press (1982), 1-12.

Bodana, A. Antimutagenic activity of milk fermented by *Streptococcus thermophilus* and *Lactobacillus bulgaricus*. Journal of Dairy Science (1990) 73(12): 3379-84.

Borriello SP, Hammes WP, et al. Safety of probiotics that contain lactobacilli or bifidobacteria. Clin Infect Dis (2003) 36:775-80.

Bosch JA, Brand HS, et al. Psychological stress as a determinant of protein levels and salivary-induced aggregation of *Streptococcus gordonii* in human whole saliva. Psychosom Med (1996) 58: 374-82.

Bosch JA, Ring C, et al. Stress and secretory immunity. Int Rev Neurobiol (2002) 52; 213-253.

Bosch JA, Turkenberg M, et al. Stress as a determinant of saliva-mediated adherence and coadherence of oral and nonoral microorganisms. Psychosom Med (2003) 65: 604-612.

Brambilla E, Gagliani M, et al. The influence of light-curing time on the bacterial colonization of resin composite surfaces. Dental Materials (2009) 25: 1067-1072.

Brown LJ, Loe H. Prevalence, extent, severity and progression of periodontal disease. Periodontol (2000) 2: 57-71.

Bryant, M. The shift to probiotics. The Journal of Alternative Medicine. (1986) 2: 6-9.

Chabance B, Marteau P, et al. Casein peptide release and passage to the blood in humans during digestion of milk or yogurt. Biochimie (1998) 80:155-65.

Çaglar E, Kargul B, Tanboga I. Bacteriotherapy and probiotics' role on oral health. Oral Dis (2005) 11: 131-7.

Cannon RD, Chaffin WL. Oral colonization by *Candida albicans* . Rev Oral Biol Med (1999) 10: 359-83.

Clemmesen, J. Antitumor effect of lactobacilli substances: "*L. bulgaricus* effect." Molecular Biotherapeutic *(1989)* 1(5): 279-82.

de Vrese M, Schrezenmeir J. Probiotics and non-intestinal infectious conditions. Br J Nutr (2002) 88: Suppl 1:S59-66.

Elmer GW, Surawicz CM, McFarland LV. Biotherapeutic agents. A neglected modality for the treatment and prevention of selected intestinal and vaginal infections. JAMA (1996) 275:870-6.

Food and Agriculture Organization of the United Nations and World Health Organization Working Group Report. Regulatory and clinical aspects of dairy probiotics. FAO and WHO Expert Consultation Report (2001). (Online)

Kekkonen RA, Lummela N, et al. Probiotic intervention has strain-specific anti-inflammatory effects in healthy adults. World J Gastroenterol (2008) 14 (13): 2029-2036.

Levine MJ. Salivary macromolecules. A structure/function synopsis. Ann NY Acad Sci (1993) 694: 11-16.

Lin, M. Antioxidative ability of lactic acid bacteria. Journal of Agricultural Food Chemistry (1999) 47(4): 1460-66.

Macfarlane GT, Cummings JH. Probiotics, infection and immunity. Curr Opin Infect Dis (2002) 15:501-6.

Madsen K. Probiotics and the immune response. (2006) 40: 232-4.

Metchnikoff, E. *The Prolongation of Life,*. Heinemann. (1907)

Molin G. Probiotics in foods not containing milk or milk constituents, with special reference to *Lactobacillus plantarum* 299v. Am J Clin Nutr (2001) 73(Suppl): 380S-5S.

Pasteur L, Joubert JF. Charbon et septicémie. C R Soc Biol Paris (1877) 85: 101-115.

Näse L, K. Hatakka K, et al. Effect of long-term consumption of a probiotic bacterium, *Lactobacillus rhamnosus* GG, in milk on dental caries and caries risk in children. Caries Res (2001) 35:412-420.

Petti S, Tarsitani G, D'Arca AS. A randomized clinical trial of the effect of yoghurt on the human salivary microflora. Arch Oral Biol (2001) 46 :705-12.

Pool-Zobel, B. Lactobacillus and bifidobacterium-mediated antigenotoxicity in the colon of rats. Nutrition and Cancer (1996) 26(3): 365-80.

Rasic, J. *Bifidobacteria and Their Role*. (1983) Boston: Birkhauser Verlag Publishers, Reid G,

Jass J, et al. Potential uses of probiotics in clinical practice. Clin Microbiol Rev (2003) 16: 658-672.

Rauen MS, Moreira EAM, et al. Oral condition and its relationship to nutritional status in the institutionalized elderly population. J Am Diet Assoc (2006) 106:1112-1114

Schüpbach P, Neeser JR, et al. Incorporation of caseinoglycomacro- and caseinophosphopeptide into the salivary pellicle inhibits adherence of mutans streptococci. J Dent Res (1996) 75: 1779-1788.

Shackelford, L. Effect of feeding fermented milk on the incidence of chemically induced colon tumors in rats. Nutrition and Cancer (1983) 5(3-4): 159-64.

Shahani, K. Natural antibiotic activity of *Lactobacillus acidophilus* and *bulgaricus*." Cultured Dairy Products Journal (1976) 11(4): 14-21

Tagg JR, Dierksen KP. Bacterial replacement therapy: adapting "germ warfare" to infection prevention. Trends Biotechnol (2003) 21: 217-233.

Shah NP. Effects of milk-derived bioactive: an overview. Br J Nutr (2000) 84: Suppl. 1, S3-10.

Touhami, M. Clinical consequences of replacing milk with yogurt in persistent infantile diarrhea. Annuals of Pediatics (Paris), (1992) 39(2):79-86.

6 GLOSSARY

Acceptable Daily Intake (ADI): FDA established acceptable daily intake limit of an artificial sweetener. It is calculated by dividing the body weight in pounds by 2.2 and then multiplying it by the ADI limit. The ADI limit for aspartame, for example, is 50 so that for a person weighing 200 lb (91 kg) and the ADI for aspartame would be 91 x 50 or 4550 mg.

Adipocyte: human fat cell.

Adipogenic: fat-producing.

Albuminuria: excess amount of the protein albumin in the urine, a sensitive marker for early kidney damage.

Amebicide: drug that acts on amoebae and amebic infections.

Anaerobic bacteria or anaerobes are a class of bacteria that can survive without oxygen for growth.

Aerobic bacteria (aerobes): bacteria that require oxygen to perform cellular respiration and which grow and multiply only in the presence of oxygen.

Anaerobic bacteria (anaerobes): bacteria that can survive without oxygen for their growth and multiplication.

Antibody: protein substances developed by the body in response to an antigen.

Antigen: substance that induces the formation of antibodies; antibodies provide immunity against the disease-producing agent inducing antibody formation.

Antioxidant: molecule capable of slowing or preventing the oxidation of other molecules and which can terminate chain reactions caused by free radicals formed in oxidation reactions. Antioxidants are often reducing agents such as polyphenols.

Archaea: single-celled microorganisms without a cell nucleus or other organelles within their cells.

Atopic dermatitis: inflammation of the skin of unknown etiology characterized by itching and scratching.

Bacillus: rod-shaped microorganism. Also, a rod-shaped aerobic bacterium belonging to the genus *Bacillaceae*; *B.* anthracis is the causative agent of anthrax.

Bacteriocin: protein produced by certain gram-positive and gram-negative bacteria that kills sensitive micro-organisms.

Bactericidal: a drug that destroys bacteria.

Bacteriophage: (also known as a phage) a type of virus that infects bacteria by injecting genetic material. Used for over 100 years as an alternative therapy to antibiotics for bacterial infections in Russia, the former Soviet Union, Eastern Europe and France.

Bacteriostatic: a drug that inhibits bacterial growth.

<u>Bacteriotherapy</u>: also known as bacterioprophylaxis, is commonly referred to as replacement therapy and is the application of probiotics to competitively reduce levels of pathogenic bacteria.

<u>Bifidobacteria</u>: Gram-positive, non-motile, anaerobic bacteria inhabiting the gastrointestinal tract and vagina. They are one of the major genera of bacteria that reside in the colon. Before the 1960s, *Bifidobacterium* species were collectively referred to as "*Lactobacillus bifidus*".

<u>Bifidogenic factor</u>: any component of the diet that stimulates the growth of bifidobacteria.

<u>Biosystem</u>: comprehensive term for the human body and its various component organs and systems.

<u>BLIS</u>: bacteriocin-like inhibitory substances produced by certain micro-organisms.

<u>BMI (body-mass index</u>): common but imperfect gauge of whether an individual is over- or underweight. BMI is the ratio of weight in kilograms to the square of height in meters. A

person who is 5ft 6inches tall with a weight of 100lb has a BMI of 16.2 while a 5ft 6inch person weight 150 lb. has a BMI of 24.2.

Bright's disease: a form of nephritis or kidney disease characterized by albumin in the urine.

Caffeine: xanthine alkaloid that is a psychoactive stimulant drug through its effect on the central nervous system.

Camellia sinensis: the tea plant.

Casein: the principal protein in milk and milk products.

Caseinopeptides: peptides derived from casein.

Catechins: polyphenols present in tea and coffee.

CFU: colony-forming unit, a measure of the numbers of viable bacterial or fungal species. The results commonly are expressed as CFU/mL (colony-forming units per milliliter) in liquids and CFU/g (colony-forming units per gram) in solids.

Chemotherapy: treatment of disease by the administration of drugs.

Chyme: mixture of partly digested food and digestive secretions found in the stomach and small intestine during digestion of foodstuffs.

Coccus (plural: cocci): spherical or ovoid-shaped bacterium.

Colitis: inflammation of the colon.

Collagen: fibrous protein found in connective tissue, including skin, bone cartilage and ligaments.

Commensal: two or more organisms that exist in an intimate but non-parasitic relationship.

Constipation: a condition characterized by bowel movements that are infrequent or hard to pass; constipation is also known costiveness as well as by the medical terms dyschezia, and dyssynergic defecation.

Cortisol: adrenal cortical hormone (the pharmaceutical product is known as hydrocortisone); also known as the stress hormone.

Crohn's disease: a perpetual gut inflammation by the immune system

CRP (C-Reactive Protein): a special type of protein produced in the liver that is present in serum during episodes of acute inflammation or infection.

Diastolic: Pertaining to the diastole or period in the heart cycle when the heart relaxes and dilates and the cavities fill with blood. Diastolic pressure is the lower number in blood pressure measurements.

Diploid: having the basic chromosome number doubled.

Disease: an abnormality of structure or function with an identifiable pathological basis and which has a recognizable constellation of clinical signs and/or a condition that is identifiable by chemical, hematological, microbiological, biophysical or immunological means.

Diverticulitis: inflammation of diverticula in the intestinal tract, especially the colon.

Diverticulosis: defects in the weakened walls of the colon and intestines due to presence of diverticula (abnormally protruding sacs or pouches).

Dysbiosis: overgrowth of bad bacteria and yeast in the intestinal tract.

EFSA: European Food Standards Authority.

EGCG (epigallocatechin-3-gallate): principal anti-oxidant catechin in green tea.

Elastin: protein that constitutes about 30% of yellow elastic tissue.

Endemic disease: a physical disorder caused by health conditions constantly present within a community and the term commonly applies to an infection transmitted directly or indirectly between humans and which occurs at the usual expected rate.

Endogenous: produced or arising within a cell or an organism.

Endotoxin: bacterial toxin within the body of a bacterium that is freed only when the bacterium breaks down.

Enzyme: organic catalyst produced by living cells; enzymes are complex proteins that catalyze chemical changes in other substances without undergoing change themselves. Many enzymes have the suffix *ase* indicating the substance they act upon, e.g. acetylcholinesterase breaks down acetylcholine.

Enzyme mediated reactions: enzymes catalyze chemical reactions that otherwise might occur too slowly to sustain life, e.g. oxidation of organic foodstuffs to provide energy. Some enzymes accelerate biochemical reactions by a factor of a thousand or more.

Epigenic: related to the theory that parts of an organism arise through progressive development from simple to complex structures by using cells as building units as opposed to the theory that parts exist preformed in the ovum or egg.

Ergogenic effect: improvement in, typically, athletic performance due to stimulants such as caffeine.

ESCF: European Scientific Committee on Food.

Eubiosis: balance between beneficial and pathogenic bacteria within the gastrointestinal tract.

Exogenous: originating outside an organ or the body.

FAO: Food and Agriculture Organization of the United Nations

FDA: U.S. Food and Drug Administration.

FSA: UK Food Standards Agency.

Facultative: the ability of a bacterium to live with or without a specific agent such as oxygen.

Flatulence: excessive gas in the stomach and intestines.

Flatus: gas in the digestive tract.

Flora: plant life occurring, or adapted to living, in a specific environment, for example, intestinal flora; in this context, flora more appropriately describes bacterial species.

Fructan: a polymer of fructose molecules. Short chain length fructans are known as fructooligosaccharides, whereas longer chain fructans are termed inulins.

Fructokinase: an enzyme of the liver, intestine, and kidney cortex. Its main role is in sucrose and fructose metabolism.

Fructooligosaccharide: a short chain of fructose molecules; also known as oligofructose or oligofructan.

Fructose: a simple monosaccharide found in many foods that is also known as levulose. Significant amounts of fructose are present as the fructose derivative sucrose (table sugar) in honey, tree fruits, berries, melons, and some root vegetables. It has the same empirical formula as glucose. Crystalline fructose and high-fructose corn syrup are often confused as the same substance. The former is often produced from a fructose-enriched corn syrup and is a true monosaccharide.

Fungicide: agent or drug that acts against fungi and fungal infections.

Gastroenterology: study of the physiology and pathology of the stomach, intestines and related structures.

<u>Gastrointestinal (GI)</u>: refers to the digestive tract.

<u>Glycogen</u>: large, branched polymer of linked glucose residues (portions of larger molecules) and is the principal storage form of glucose in animal cells, and is also found in various bacteria and fungi.

<u>Gram's Method</u>: a method for staining bacteria and is important in identifying bacteria.

<u>Gram-negative</u>: a bacterium that loses the stain and adopts the color of the counter stain in Gram's staining method.

<u>Gram-positive</u>: a bacterium that retains the color of the gentian violet stain used in Gram's staining method.

<u>Haploid</u>: possessing half the diploid or number of chromosomes found in body cells.

<u>High-fructose corn syrup</u>: a mixture of nearly equal amounts of fructose and glucose.

<u>Homeostasis</u>: state of equilibrium of the internal environment of the body.

<u>Hypomotility</u>: slow transit of digesta through the colon.

Immunoglobulin: proteins capable of acting as antibodies, five major types of which are known.

Indigenous: native to a country, region or the human biosystem.

Inulin: a longer chain fructan or polysaccharide composed of a heterogeneous blend of polymerized fructofuranose (fructose) units; stimulates intestinal bifidobacteria

Irritable bowel syndrome: altered bowel habits (e.g. constipation, diarrhea, bloating, abdominal pain, cramping and spasm) caused not by a disease but by various factors such as stress and anxiety, poor diet and various medications.

Lactoferricin: a peptide with anti-microbial and anti-cancer properties generated by the pepsin-mediated digestion of lactoferrin.

Lactoferrin: also known as lactotransferrin, a protein with antimicrobial (bactericidal and fungicidal) activity found in milk and mucosal secretions such as tears and saliva.

<u>Lactoperoxidase:</u> an <u>enzyme</u> secreted from mammary, salivary and other mucosal glands that functions as a natural antibacterial agent.

<u>Lactose</u>: a disaccharide <u>sugar</u> formed from <u>galactose</u> and <u>glucose</u> that makes up 2~8% of milk by weight, although the actual content varies between species and individuals.

<u>Leukopenia:</u> decrease in the number of white blood cells (leukocytes) in the blood, placing individuals at increased risk of infection.

<u>Ligand</u>: an entity that binds to a complex central ion or to a substrate.

<u>Lipoprotein:</u> conjugated (coupled together) proteins consisting of simple proteins combined with lipids (fats), e.g. cholesterol and triglycerides.

<u>Lymphadenopathy</u>: disease of the lymph nodes, a term used almost synonymously with swollen or enlarged lymph nodes.

<u>Mesentery</u>: peritoneal fold encircling most of the small intestines and connecting them to the posterior abdominal wall.

Methylxanthines: methylated derivatives of xanthine; they include caffeine and theobromine which are present in coffee and tea.

Micellar: adjective based on a micelle, a submicroscopic unit of protoplasm built up from polymer molecules or a colloidal aggregate of 50-100 certain types of molecules.

Minimum inhibitory concentration (MIC): of an antibacterial is the maximum dilution of that drug that will still inhibit the growth of a test microorganism.

Morbid: affected by disease; related to or characteristic of disease.

Morbidity: state of being diseased or the number of persons affected by a disease within a specific population.

Motility: ability to move spontaneously, e.g. digesta through the intestinal tract.

Murein: (also known as peptidoglycan) is a polymer consisting of sugars and amino acids that forms a mesh-like layer surrounding the plasma membrane of bacteria, forming the cell wall.

Naturopathy: therapeutic system that uses natural forces such as light, heat, air, water and massage for patient treatment rather than drugs.

Neutropenia: hematological disorder characterized by an abnormally low number of neutrophils, the most important type of white blood cell.

Nitric oxide (NO): an important messenger molecule involved in many physiological (and pathological) processes. It is a signaling molecule often involved in transmitting information between cells by interacting with receptors in another cell to trigger a response in that cell.

Nosocomial: hospital acquired, as in nosocomial infections.

Obligate: e.g. an obligate aerobe is a bacterium that must have oxygen in order to live.

Oligo: scientific term for a few.

Oligodynamic effect: toxic effect of metal-ions on living cells and microorganisms, even in relatively low concentrations. This antimicrobial effect is shown by ions of silver and copper as well as other metals such as zinc, iron, gold, aluminum, iron and bismuth. Bacteria (Gram-positive and Gram-negative) are in general affected by the oligodynamic effect but can develop a heavy-metal resistance. Viruses in general are poorly sensitive.

Oligofructose: a subgroup of inulin, consisting of polymers with up to 10 polymer units; stimulates intestinal bifidobacteria.

Oligosaccharide: a short chain of sugar molecules consisting of 2-8 monosaccharide units linked by glycoside bonds; also known as compound sugar.

Organelle: part of a cell that performs a definite function.

Oxidation: chemical reaction in which electrons are transferred from a substance to an oxidizing agent; oxidation reactions can produce free radicals which can initiate chain reactions that damage cells.

<u>pH</u>: the pH of an aqueous solution is a measure of its acidity or basicity (alkalinity) and is based on the hydrogen ion (H^+) activity in solution. Pure water is neutral, with a pH close to 7.0, whereas solutions with a pH less than 7 (pH < 7.0) are acidic and those with a pH greater than 7 (pH > 7.0) are basic or alkaline.

<u>Pathogenic</u>: disease-causing

<u>Pathogenicity</u>: propensity for causing disease.

<u>Pepsin</u>: primary enzyme of gastric juice that digests proteins.

<u>Peptides</u>: substances prepared by synthesis from amino acids that are intermediate in chemical properties and molecular weight between amino acids and proteins.

<u>Peptidoglycan</u>: (also known as murein) is a polymer consisting of sugars and amino acids that forms a mesh-like layer surrounding the plasma membrane of bacteria, that is, the polymer serves a structural role in the bacterial cell wall by conferring strength on the structure.

Peritoneum: serum-producing membrane covering the viscera and lining the abdominal cavity.

Phenylketonuria (PKU): disease caused by the body's failure to oxidize the amino acid phenylalanine, possibly because of a defective enzyme. The incidence is 1: 40, 000 births in the U.S. and 1: 25,000 births in the UK.

Plasma: liquid part of the lymph and blood.

Polyphenols: a group of chemical substances, commonly antioxidants, found in plants which contain two or more phenol units per molecule; they are divided into the hydrolysable tannins (e.g. tannic acid) and other sugars, and phenylpropanoids, such as lignins, flavonoids, and condensed tannins.

Polysaccharide: name given to any member of a class of relatively complex, high-molecular weight carbohydrates consisting of long-chains of many monosaccharides (sugars) joined together. Well-known polysaccharides include starch, glycogen, cellulose and chitin.

Prebiotic: selectively fermented food ingredient that beneficially affects the host through specific stimulation of the growth and/or activity of one or more bacteria in the colon.

Probiotic: foodstuff containing a live microbiological culture

Prokaryotes: group of organisms that lack a cell nucleus (or karyon) or any other membrane-bound organelles.

Proteolytic activity: ability to split proteins and facilitate their digestion and absorption by the host.

Protista: simplest organisms that are acellular or unicellular, and include bacteria, spirochetes, some algae, protozoa and other life forms not readily classified as either animals or plants.

Pyrogenesic: causing a fever.

Ribonucleic acid (RNA): nucleic acid found in certain cell components and has an important role in synthesizing reactions within cells.

Ribosome: extremely small portion of the submicroscopic cell structure containing ribonucleoprotein and synthesizes protein.

Rotavirus: most common cause of severe diarrhea among infants and young children but rarely affects adults. Virtually all children have been infected with rotavirus at least once by the age of five although immunity develops with each succeeding infection, and subsequent infections are less severe. Five species of the virus are known, Types A through E, with rotavirus A being the most common and causing > 90% of infections.

Saccharide: scientific term for a sugar.

Serum: watery portion of blood after coagulation; injectable animal-derived serum consists of plasma without fibrinogen.

Sjögren's syndrome: auto-immune disease that causes damage to fluid-producing glands such as the tear ducts and saliva glands, resulting in dry mouth and eyes.

<u>Sucrose</u>: a disaccharide derived from the condensation of glucose and fructose. Sucrose, commonly known as table sugar, is formed by plants but not other organisms.

<u>Synbiotic</u>: combination of a prebiotic and probiotic in a single product.

<u>Systolic</u>: pertaining to the systole or contraction of the heart when blood is forced through the circulatory system. Systolic pressure is the upper number in blood pressure measurements.

<u>Tannic acid</u>: polyphenol comprising glucose esters of gallic acid.

<u>Telemores</u>: the DNA sequences at the end of chromosomes, i.e. the "end filler" of human DNA strands. Telemores shorten with aging and when consumed, the cell is destroyed. Some scientists believe that telomeres, and telomerase the enzyme which controls the lengthening/shortening of telomeres on human DNA, are key to aging and cancer.

<u>Theaflavin</u>: antioxidant polyphenols formed from catechins in tea leaves during the enzymatic

oxidation (or fermentation) of the leaves during preparation of black tea.

Theanine: an amino acid commonly found in tea.

Theobromine: an alkaloid of the cacao plant, found in chocolate and in many chocolate-free foods made from theobromine sources including the leaves of the tea plant; it has a similar, but lesser, effect to caffeine.

Urticaria: allergic reaction marked by skin rash, e.g. nettle rash and hives.

Viricide: agent or drug that acts on viruses.

WHO: the World Health Organization

Xanthine: a purine base found in most body tissues and fluids; mild stimulants such as caffeine and theobromine are derived from xanthine.

J. A. von FRAUNHOFER

ABOUT THE AUTHOR

Dr. J. Anthony von Fraunhofer is Professor Emeritus, University of Maryland, Baltimore. He studied at Sir John Cass College, University of London where he was awarded a BSc degree with honors in chemistry and gained his MSc and PhD degrees. He has Chartered Scientist, Chartered Chemist and Chartered Engineer designations from the United Kingdom Science Council. He holds Fellowships in the Academy of Dental Materials, ASM International, the Institute of Corrosion and the Royal Society of Chemistry.

After several years in industrial R&D, Dr. von Fraunhofer joined the Institute of Dental Surgery, University of London as a Lecturer before being promoted to Senior Lecturer and Chairman of the

Department of Biomaterials Science. He was recruited to the Health Sciences Center, University of Louisville in 1978 and moved to the University of Maryland, Baltimore in 1994.

Dr. von Fraunhofer has mentored 14 Ph.D. and 120 M.S. degree candidates, and written over 400 scientific papers, 13 books, and contributed chapters to 12 monographs. He has made over 140 research presentations at National/International meetings and lectured and presented courses in the United States, England, Continental Europe, North Africa and the Middle East. His fields of interest include physical and mechanical properties of biomaterials; dental cutting; wound closure devices and wound healing; degradation, wear and corrosion of materials in the biosystem as well as in industrial applications. He also holds a number of patents in the field of biomaterials science.

Printed in Great Britain
by Amazon.co.uk, Ltd.,
Marston Gate.